Life is Hard
Life is Beautiful

May you find glimmers of Beauty even through life's Hard times.
— Janell Meier

Janell Meier

Copyright © 2024 by Janell Meier.

All rights reserved. No part of this publication may be reproduced, distributed or transmitted in any form or by any means, including photocopying, recording, or other electronic or mechanical methods, without the prior written permission of the publisher, except in the case of brief quotations embodied in critical reviews and certain other noncommercial uses permitted by copyright law. For permission requests, write to the author, at: janellmeier@gmail.com.

Author
Janell Meier

Photographers
Janell Meier
Audrey Werlinger "Authentic"
Barb Tholkes "Story"

Publisher
Janell Meier

Website
janellmeier.com

Life is Hard Life is Beautiful / Janell Meier —1st ed.
ISBN 979-8-9912880-0-2

This book is dedicated to those who are hurting through life's hard times. My hope is that this book will help you feel less alone.

To my B & B, my rock and my hope. This is for you. A tangible legacy of how hard times can also lead us to beauty. The beauty you provide me every single day has never been lost on me.

Contents

Introduction 6

I. Life is Hard 8

Night	10
Wilted	11
I Know	12
I Learned	13
Stage 4 Ocean	14
Maiden	18
Crone	20
Hope	21
Now	22
Challenge	23
Flame	24
Air	25
Yesterday	26
Tomorrow	27
Someday	28
Time	29
Fear	30
Enough	31
Live	32
Listen	33
Real Life?	34
Strings	36
Step	37
But Then	38

II. Life is Beautiful 40

Whisper	42
Shout	43
Grasp	44
Create	45
Anticipation	46
Begin	48
Music	50
Play	51
Wisdom	52
Identity	53
Wonder	54
Wander	55
Ripple	56
Disco Balls	57
Seed	58
Waiting	59
Water	60
Growth	62
Harvest	63
Taste	64
Year-End	65
Reflection	66

III. Life is Hard and Beautiful 68

Dear Younger Self 70
Time Stamped Moments 71
Story 72
Story: Part 2 73
Living Room 74
Touch 76
Overwhelmed 78
Overwhelmed Reframed 79
Belong 80
Even In 81
Authentic 82
Expectation 83
Writing 84
The Timeless Moment 85
What Matters 86
Dear Cancer 88

IV. Reflect and Write 90

Your Mind 92
Place 94
Learn 96
Grief 98
Joy 100
Dash 102
Reframe 104

Introduction

I was inspired to write this book because I recognize the pain and beauty of life. I know we all have, or will face, difficult life circumstances. Through my more challenging times, I have found that picking up a pen or opening my computer and filling a blank page brought out so many thoughts and emotions that I did not know I was holding. Writing became a way to process what was happening in my life. Then, I found that sharing my pieces with others brought another level of healing.

Often I could not explain my feelings or articulate my experiences. But when I allowed myself the space and gifted myself with a blank page, things would become clearer in just a few minutes.

When I was diagnosed with breast cancer at the age of 27 I was fortunate in that I was young, strong, and otherwise healthy. This mindset helped me stay positive through chemotherapy treatment. However, I did not allow myself much opportunity at that time to grieve all the ways cancer was affecting my life.

Years later I was finally able to sit with the pain that came with all the ways cancer broke my body and relationships, including putting on hold my dream of becoming a mother. This book is a compilation of the many emotions of my life and how I learned to gain perspective from more than one side of my experiences.

I intentionally organized this book so that it can be opened and enjoyed in any order. I do have separate sections for when your life might feel hard or beautiful. You can search the topics within those sections to find poems to meet you where you are at, in any given moment. There are prompts and space in the back of the book as an open invitation should you feel inspired to write your own words. I would love for you to pick up a pen and explore your life circumstances.

My wish is for these words to help you feel less alone. My vulnerability here has provided me strength, and often hope. May it do the same for you.

~ ~ ~ ~

This book is meant to offer inspiration for healing and growth. It is not a substitute for mental health professionals. Please be aware that this book includes sensitive topics including: cancer, death, and grief.

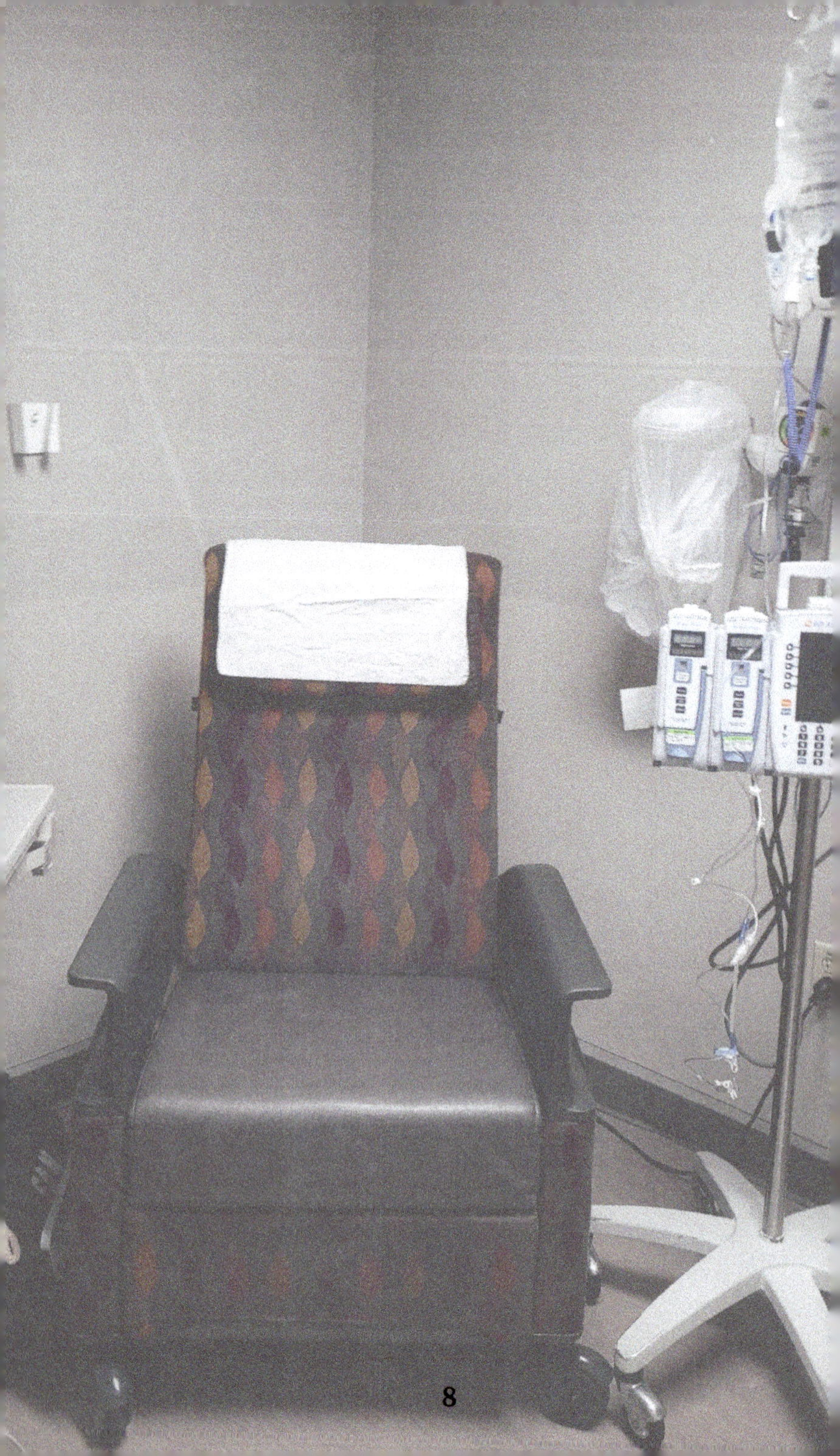

Life is Hard

*May you find healing
in the words that follow*

Night

After the sun sets
when the sky turns
the color of lost hope

Then, slowly stars begin to appear

The sky's magic
seems a little closer

The moon
lights the darkened path

Enough to move forward

Wilted

The beauty I remember
The flickers
    knowing
    and
    unknowing
That this will change my life forever

Past the fleeting childhood
Camping with cousins
Bike rides and softball games
Lacing up my hockey skates

Moving to campus
Meeting the man I'd marry
Dreaming of the future

Blindsided by the biopsy call

Wilted into a world unknown

Writing to withstand it all

I Know

I don't know exactly what you're going through, but

I know how it feels to hear those words from the doctor

I know what it feels like to wait

I know the feeling of
   plans being interrupted
   of wanting to be strong for everyone else

I know what it feels like
   to be a burden

I know what it's like to

                            worry

                                  wonder

                                      wait

I Learned

What I learned was
    I am Worthy of love

I learned to
    lean in, even when I wanted to run
    let go, even when my fists were clenched tight
    accept help, even when I wanted to walk alone

I learned to take one day, one hour, at a time

It helped me to
    plan something exciting
    while being flexible to possible changes

I learned to gain strength and wisdom
from others on similar paths
who were ready to offer support

Over time, I learned
crying sometimes helps

So does keeping a routine and
being surrounded by those I love

What I learned was
    I can survive hard times
    Strength looks different each day
    Courage is continuing on,
    even when fear is staring you down

Stage 4 Ocean

A whirlwind of emotions
within a few short hours.
The camaraderie of best friends.
Showing up for scans
within minutes of each other.

We sit together and wait
for our names to be called;
for the scans that will determine our future.

After, going to breakfast with our husbands,
who are riding this wave with us
in this ocean we call Stage 4.

Hours later,
at the same time,
the four of us sit
in two different rooms.

We hear the results from that morning.
I hear my results and see the scans.
The doctor leaves the room briefly.
I want to celebrate.
I want to thank God
for my answered prayers
– results far beyond
human understanding or belief.

I text her, my soul sister.
She responds
"progression".

In our Stage 4 ocean
this means a storm
is pushing you from the shore
you want so desperately
to land your feet upon,
even if just for
a few minutes.

The one word from her leaves me feeling sick.
As tears of guilt roll down my face
I'm left questioning
Why?
Why are my prayers answered? Hers not?
Why are we here at the same time, same hour?
Why can't we both get good news?

She's brought me so much life.

I owe her
for playing a huge part in bringing us our
miracle baby.
I owe her for pushing me to get the scan
that revealed my stage 4 diagnosis.
I owe her.

Yet, today, there is
nothing
I can do
for her.

We both sit in our vessels,
side by side.
We continue riding the waves,
as we look around,
searching for the
lighthouse.

This time
I wish I could
pull her to shore
with me.

And I know, in the past, she's felt
the same way for me.

Our hearts break
for each other
with each diagnosis;
with each scan
    we hold our breaths
        and submerge
            into the ocean
until the results are in.

All that I know to do is
pray.
Pray that this new treatment
works better for her
than the last.
Pray that another miracle is given,
next time to my dear
soul sister.

I know she will
continue her fight,
as will I.
We will fight on.

We will celebrate the victories
and curse the waves that knock us down
along the way.
We will live each day
to the best of our abilities.

And most importantly,
we will be there for each other,
as sisters always are.

Maiden

Back to the maiden days
 when my world was wild and free
 when I was to create myself
  and my future.

Like the destructive swirling of a
 Midwest summer tornado

There is so much to consider and choose.
What if these choices leave a path
 of total destruction?

Some choices heavy, like a fallen
 tree on top of a house.
The "right" choice feels like finding
 a blade of grass
 stuck in a tree trunk
 after the dirt settles.

How do I know? How do I trust?

I can look back now,
    confident each choice shaped
        where I am.
No wrong choices.
      All stepping stones
      to today.

My maturity has allowed me
    to look back and appreciate
    all the paths along the way.
I know now, I can trust the future,
    the choices aren't all on my
    shoulders.
I know now, there's not one right way.

Choose your own adventures in life.
You'll be okay.

Crone
Caught between two worlds
Thrown into Crone
        while wishing to
                embrace Motherhood
So much lost
looking at life
        in this warped reality
Now wise
        feeling robbed of the
                beauty
                and simplicity
                of Mother
Living far too close
to the edge of Crone
                Wanting to live joyfully
but watching my back
for what could be lurking
                Celebrating each birthday,
                  both my baby's and mine,
yet counting each candle,
wondering if, for me,
it'll be the last cake
of its time
        Time - grateful for each moment
yet cursing
the Crone
inside me
        who understands
          the fragility of
                Woman.

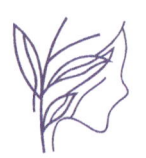

HOPE

H – Hold
O – On
P – Persevere, keep Perspective
E – Enjoy life and all it offers

Now

Someday

I'll see you again

Someday

I'll meet you there

In those last moments you gave me a
Strength and Faith
    I didn't know I could hold

Someday
    I stopped fearing death,
    though still scared to leave,
    I am learning
    that I am Here

making Someday's
                  moments
                            now.

Challenge

A challenge:
    That difficult semester-end test
    A high school fight with your best friend
    Feeling alone in the full halls of school

Hearing the words: you have cancer
    Putting life into perspective
    Doctor appointments, procedures, surgeries
Hearing the words: you beat cancer
    Going to prom
    Getting ready for college

Only to hear that "C" word again
    Instead of college
        it's the cancer floor of the hospital
    Instead of exams
        it's medical scans and medications

A life challenge like no other
    A challenge that took your life far too soon

Not the future you or your family chose
    But it was carried and transformed
    Into a legacy
        That changed my life
        Because of your courage

    And for that, I am forever grateful

Flame

The fire burns deep
yet one sprinkle of water
    one doubt inside
and I let it die away

What is it I fear with the fire?

Why can't I flame the fire to burn bright?

With a small movement I could create
    big flames

Yet every time I get close
I let it
    sizzle out for something new

Air

We need it to stay alive
but rarely think about its power.
Are we grateful for it?
Speak or praise it?

Those who struggle for it,
can't think of much else.

Similar to the days following
my cancer diagnosis,
it felt disease would consume my every hour.
Over time I learned
how to sit still, nothing but my breath.
At first, forced rest –
the hour before my PET scan
or when attached to my infusion pole.

Many of us forget
each breath of air is a gift.

Like floating in a balloon basket over the
mountains at sunrise.
Or watching the sunset spread like smoke
into the ocean within minutes.

Each breath of air
is a gift.

Yesterday

Yesterday
    When days were busy
    And minutes were fleeting

Yesterday
    When the world was promised to us
    When we didn't know
        the days were numbered

Yesterday
    When life felt
        hard absurd difficult
    Little did we know then
    what a blessing

    Yesterday
    was

Yesterday
    A memory made
    Joy in the simplicity
    A new appreciation

Gained through the
new normal
learned from

    Today

Tomorrow

Tomorrow
    We wait for it
    Some with excited anticipation
    Some with dreaded fear

We wonder what might be
When we close our eyes
    What will await
    When we open them again
We put things off
    For someday
We chase what we think
    Will bring us happiness

All the while
    The reality is
    Each day is
        Another
            Tomorrow
Slipping through our grasp

Tomorrow can be
        Everything
          Nothing
              Suddenly yesterday.

Someday

Someday I'll be
    Done with school
    Married
    Buying a home

Someday I'll
    Be a Mommy
    Find a new career

Someday I'll say goodbye to my best friend

Someday I'll publish my book

Someday we'll blink
    And it'll all be through

Live for someday
    Time will pass either way

Time

A Joker
A Magician
A Genie in a bottle

We beg for more
Yet it passes the same

I fear the future
Set it aside

I scold the past
Let it go

I neglect the present
Behold it

Fear

It consumes my mind
paralyzes me

Wandering thoughts of
all that might be

Scenes in my head create
stories complex and coiled

Real
        Raw
                Rigid

How to Clear
          Create
                  Communicate?

Over time I learn
    the courage it takes
    to step out
    to trust
        that there is more
        than my Fear

Enough

What is enough?
How do I measure it?
When will my efforts
            be enough?

E - Ever trying
N - Never living up
O - Outing myself
U - Under celebrating my wins
G - Going all in without listening to my body
H - Holding on to perfectionism

Enough!
   I'm declaring now
   I've had enough, with the feeling
   of being enough.
   I am enough as is, where I am,
   with what I'm doing.

Like one pine tree
in the forest on a mountain cliff,
   I am enough.
   It's not up to me to be the forest.

I am one tree.
Without me, the forest wouldn't be full
but alone, I cannot fill the forest.

Live

As day breaks
    over the quiet dark sky

Acknowledgment that we are alive
    starting a new day
For all that might be

We live
    but do we appreciate
    just what that means

We live
    to rush to run
    to cry to plead
For another day
For another moment
We Live

As the sun sets
    before us

Do we wish for more,
    or do we accept what is,
    with peace of what was?

Listen

Listen not only to the words spoken

But to the soul of the speaker

Hear what is not said

Listen to the silence

Listen to the words of anger and despair
    Don't take them personally
    But reply with love
    Reply with grace

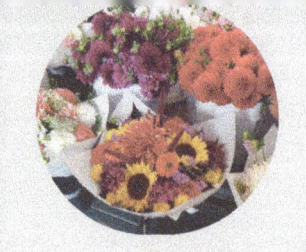

Real Life?

I open my eyes and look around
Is this a dream?
> The machines, the IVs
> The chill in the air
Is this real life?

I feel as if I haven't rested in months
Is this a dream?
> The call
> Yet again
> But this time the words dig deeper
Is this real life?

I stare at the text on my phone
Is this a dream?
> Words that appear from you
> But telling me you're gone
> News that remade me
Is this real life?

I voice my needs as I honor you
Is this a dream?
> Walking away from security
> From what no longer serves me
Is this real life?

In honoring you I create space
Is this a dream?
    Not knowing then
    But unfolding within months
    Helping our soul sister when needed most
Is this real life?

I join her at appointments
Is this a dream?
    We've done this many times before
    The tone and message different now
Is this real life?

She is given just months to live
Is this a dream?
    It's not lost on me
    Lessons learned from you
    Carried to the next experience
Is this real life?

I want to awake
Is this a dream?
    Lost hope
    Months bleed down to weeks
    Weeks and days turn to hours
Is this real life?

Is this a dream?
Is this a nightmare?
Is this real life?

Strings

The guitar strings hold our story
    I hear the depth
    I feel the suffering

Moments of beauty
among the dark chords

He creates
in honor of us
    taking on the pain
    processing it into art

Organizing the orchestra
Putting your story to lyrics

To show his love, our love,
This song will *love* on

To comfort
To remember the best friend you were to many

Step

I see the staircase
I don't know how I'll climb it
Yet I know
to have a full satisfied rest
    I must climb
    one foot in front of the other

That small and narrow staircase
    is part of a two-story house
        in a small community
            part of a small state
                within the country
    the country just a piece of our world
    our world a speck in the galaxy

I must remind myself it's just a few steps

Then I will awake
and do it all over tomorrow

One step at a time

But Then

I get her out the door for the bus
I should move my body, walk.
   But then,

I curl back into bed
just for twenty more minutes
my alarm goes off
   But then,

A headache is starting now
I should get out of bed
and pour myself coffee
   But then,

I have things to get done today
bills to pay
laundry to wash
   But then,

I know I feel better
if I move

But it's as if the
weight of the
world sits
    HEAVY
upon me

The sun is shining
winter will be here soon
I should soak up the air while it's warm
    But
      Then

I sit.
I feel.
I put pen to paper.
I lean in to what I wish I could avoid.
I tell myself
    I am enough.
I let myself be.

I name the Sadness and Grief.

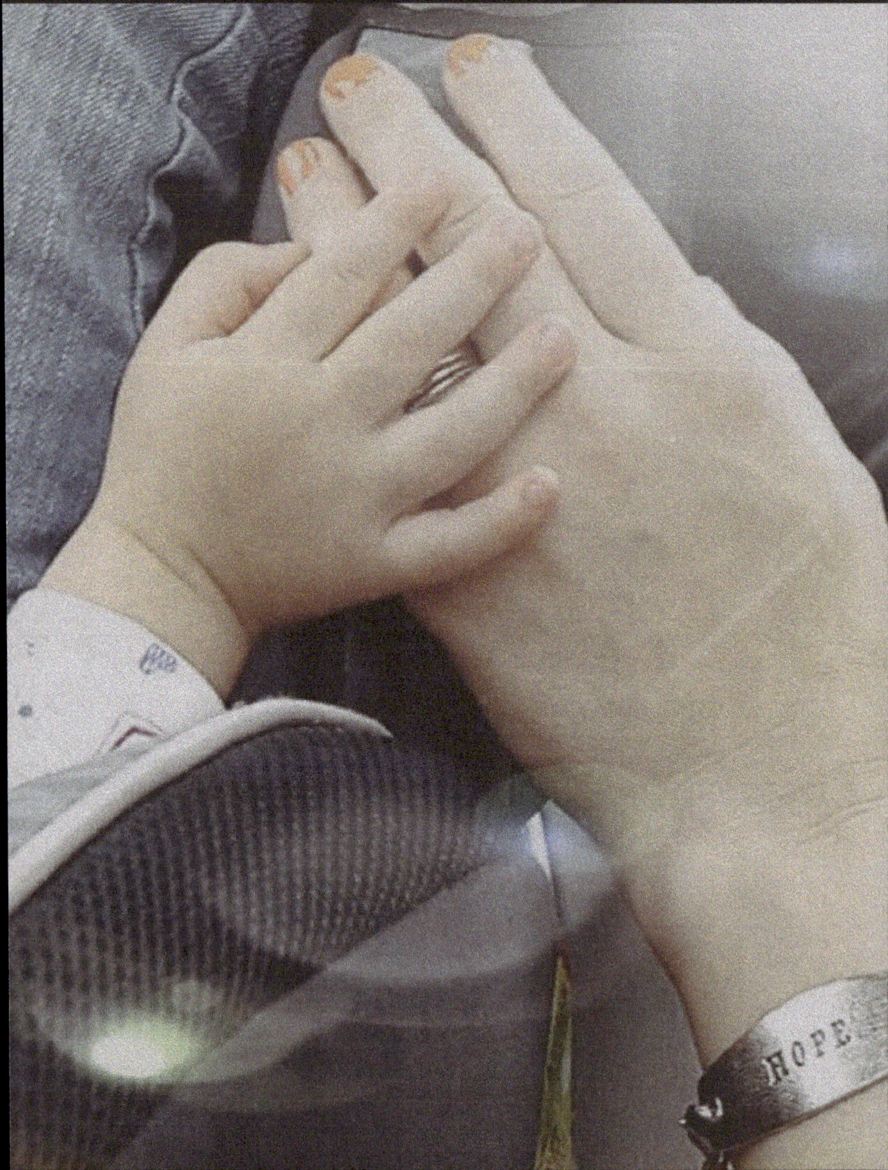
HOPE

Life is Beautiful

*May you find growth
in the words that follow*

Whisper

I arrive
It was the whisper
    That I used to ignore

I walk up the steps

These schoolhouse walls
    Will hold us for the weekend

It's the whisper
I need right now

To hear the strength within
To be at ease
To gain peace and grace

That I will carry back
And whisper to others
    That there is another way
    To arrive
        In life

Shout

The mighty water falls
   The skies crash between lightning

The lions roar
   And the wildebeests stampede

The volcano erupts
   Spewing lava and destruction

The sounds of many
   Shouting what is known

We demand to be heard
   For if the voice is strong
   Surely others will listen

But what if
   What if all was still
   What if all came together
      In a moment

      Of silence

Grasp

She doesn't grasp
    how much it means to me that
    I am here
She doesn't grasp
    how proud
    I am of her

As I grasp her tight
    she lets go
    to fly with her friends

May she always
    keep that sparkle for life
    keep that jump in her step
    keep her open heart

Create

Start with a dab of paint
    an idea
    an image
    gaze into the open sky

Create what's wanted
    what's needed
    for the soul

If we cannot create
    what is life?

Create to Hope
Create to Be
Create to Live

As I open my eyes
I create a new day
A list of dreams and ideas

A future

Anticipation

On the brink of something big
    looking over the edge
    taking that deep breath
    knowing a leap is needed
    yet scared of what's to come

What if?
    What if this time the risk
    isn't as safe as promised?
    What if this time
    something goes wrong?

But
What if it all goes right?
What if this time the experience is for you?

It's that feeling your stomach gets
when the roller coaster cart rolls up
Your eyes meet the passengers
that are just coming back to the station

They are laughing, smiling,
wiping the tears from their eyes
Their smiles as wide as their faces allow

Your turn now
to step forward
lock yourself into the seat
And enjoy the ride

You live for these rides

These adventures
The excitement
    Challenges, screams
    Highs and lows

You are
    Ready!

Begin

Begin
one word at a time
it takes courage
to put pen
to paper

What's written now
will forever be

Will it be
what I want?

Will the words flow
or will I question
each stroke?

Here I sit
curled up in our cozy basement
my only child on the theater seat
beside me

Both with our own space
our own magic blankets

The relaxing music she chose
playing from across the room
a quiet calm piano piece

This
    this is what makes
    my heart full

With our matching notebooks
we each write

I hear a deep sigh

Peace

Pride

Begin living
    the life you imagine
    the life you deserve
    the life you can create

I've done it
my Miracle Baby next to me
is all the proof I need
that God is leading us

Music

I turn to you when my heart needs a change
    Filling the void when nothing else can
    Meeting me where I'm at

We need you
    For an escape from our reality
    To provide moments that will outlive us

She is at ease with you
    I look up to her on the stage
    An inner confidence that shines bright

Thank you, for giving:
    me the words I couldn't find
    us the memories of freeness and fun
    her the voice she didn't know she had

Thank you, Music
For the gifts I will always cherish.

Play

Back when
Time stretched
Weeks felt like months
    Months felt like years
No responsibilities

That feeling when connected with my heart
    Nothing else matters
Lost in a world of its own
A time to
    Explore, Be, Create
To imagine, To dream

As adults
    These times are far too fleeting
        To retreat
        When hours feel like minutes
        And days feel like hours

It's those feelings,
These times,
That I live for

To Play
    Is to Live

Wisdom

It's in us all
If we're willing to
    Listen
    Lean in
    Sit still

Strength is needed to cut
    The noise
    A new path
    Fear

But the wisdom you seek
Is within you

Beware of
Following the shiny paths full of promises
Beware of
Others who try to decide your future
Beware of your mind leading too much
Your heart is wise

WISDOM

W - We can
I - Imagine
S - Seek
D - Dream
O - Outline
M - Make it happen

Identity

A longing to be heard
not by others
but for my own soul
to meet my heart.

As my identities are stripped
I can remake who I want to become.

Screaming to be heard
but what is it they want to say?
Whispering amongst each other
but is it true?

Wonder

Each month I continue to surrender
All areas of my life

I live

Excitement
and
Trepidation

Ready to jump but scared of the winds

Wanting to plan
While also wanting to create, to be

Wishing for the answers in a crystal ball
While knowing they're already inside me

Can I wander?

Wander

We take our Jeep and head out
No destination yet decided

Just the Hope of feeling Free

A simple Joy

We ride with the top down
    The wind swirling
Wandering the backroads between lakes

There's a chill
    Reminding that summer nights
    Will soon be replaced with autumn air

I see the dark clouds looming
Fearful of rain
But he assures me
As always,
That we'll be okay

The music up
My hand resting on his leg
We're lost in the rhythm and words

We're on this ride together
In this life together
Side by side

Ripple

One small drop to start

We choose our future

Unknown
Unaware then
What this ripple could be

Grateful for the small start
That seemed to have
Started the ocean waves

The welcomed changes
That affected me
And rippled to my family
To my friends

I had no idea then
What it would mean

I chose my future
The future to which I was called

Disco Balls

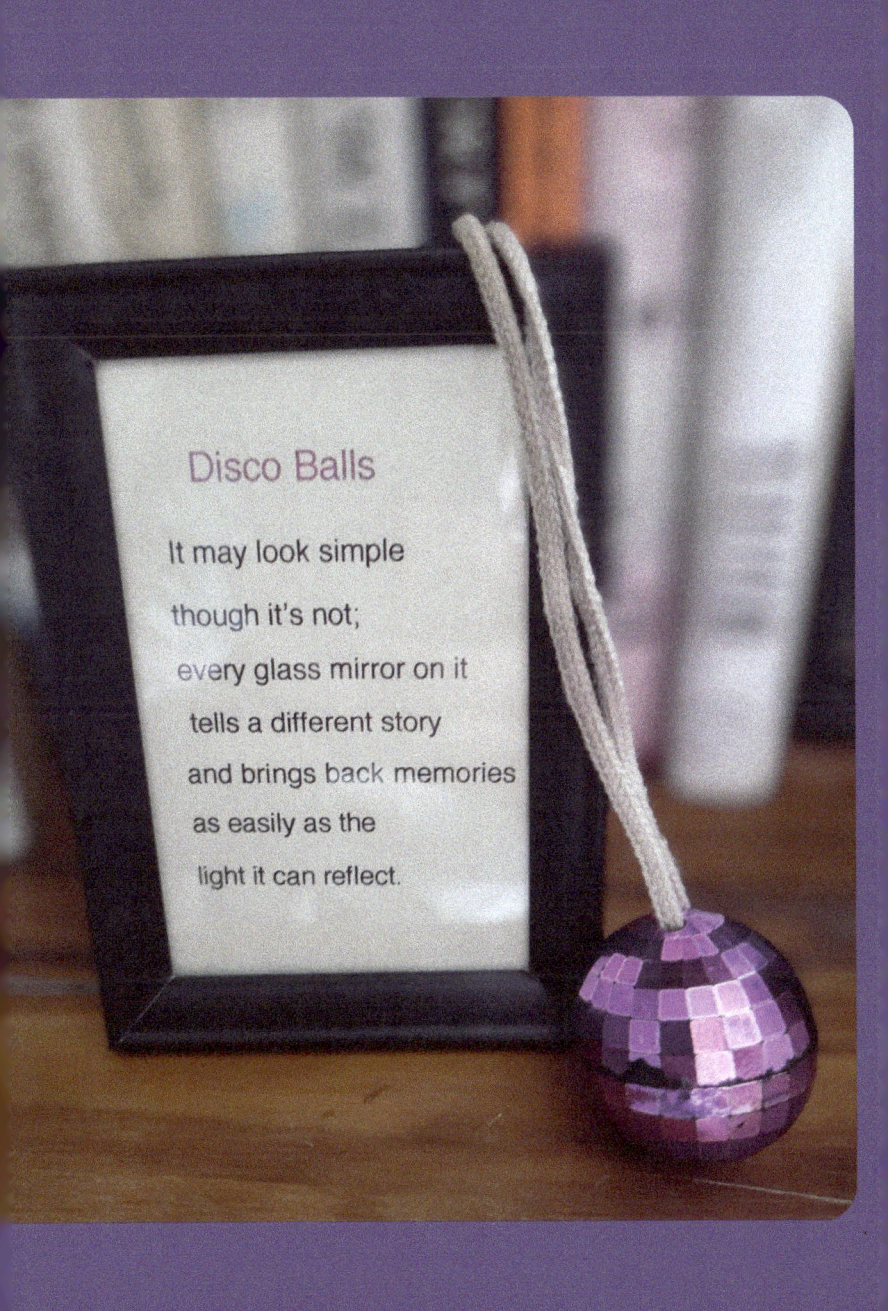

It may look simple
though it's not;
every glass mirror on it
tells a different story
and brings back memories
as easily as the
light it can reflect.

Seed

What seeds are you planting?

Each day we leave seeds
    Are yours of
        Hope, Joy, and Magic?

Or are you planting
    Fear, Resentment, and Anger?

You have the power of
    Which seeds leave your hands
    And what roots grow beneath you

One by one
    You are sprouting your own Aspen stand
Either a forest of
    Encouragement
    Idleness or darkness

If you're in the darkness, take one step towards a new grove

Slowly but surely I know you can find your way through

Waiting

Lights across the Northern still sky
Sun peeking slowly over the horizon
First sparks of a campfire

Each of us ebb and flow
We fizzle out
But then come back stronger than ever

With each seed you plant in life
Have Faith that it'll blossom
Into what is meant to be

Not all growth is noticeable
Sometimes it's necessary to
    Let the water and sun fill you first
    Sit under the night sky and take it in

Know you are meant to grow
At your own pace
With just a few resources

You have the rest within you

Waiting - Wanting - Flourishing

Water

The waves hitting the shore
Much like the 'tock' of a clock

The way standing in a steam-filled shower
    Can clear my thoughts
    And renew me

The peace that comes with
Hearing the falls
Feeling the mist kiss my cheeks
    Ever so lightly

Soaking in a tub
Floating the day's stress away

Hearing the sound of rain
Hit the house.
If I'm lucky, catching a rainbow

Floating on a Minnesota lake
Watching the sunset
And talking with my dad

Feeling the falling snow
Hit my head and hands

Sipping on hot tea
Snuggled under a blanket
Drinking the warm liquid

Splashing in the pool
Or puddles

Feeding the plants
With the same
Nourishment

I forget I long for

Water

Growth

Always putting others first
As an employee, mother, wife,
Family member, friend.

But now

Letting go
    Of guilt
    Of worth through actions

Holding tight
    To self-love
    To peace within
    To what I need

Affirming what is
Accepting life
    As it arrives
    As it unfolds

Different from what I'd expected
Doing what's necessary
Delivering the gifts I was given
So others too,
Can heal and grow

Harvest

After seeds and growth
    We get to harvest our hard work

When the moon is shining bright upon
The awaited fields aglow
When the golden crops
Are ready to retrieve
Remember you prepared for just this

Remember to harvest your workings
Don't let the nutrients lie dormant in the field
Share with those around you
Your harvest is not meant to be hoarded
Nor neglected

The harvest season
    A month
    A year
    A decade
    A lifetime

Each harvest season
    Serves its own purpose

To fill yourself
To fill your family
To fill your community
To share your knowledge with the next

Taste

I take a bite
    As I write

I eat to nourish
    But don't slow down

I want to connect
    In other ways
Forgetting that
    The bowl in front of me
    Is art too

Quinoa and kale
Sweet potatoes and beets
Pumpkin seeds and chickpeas

Each bite
    Like each word
    A savoring for my soul

Year-End

A time to reflect

A time to wrap up
    Projects, goals, plans

    Endings of chapters

        Yet life's book continues on

We put pressure and emphasis on year-end
    Yet it's another day
        Another opportunity
    To start again
    To be intentional

Building on past endings
We transform once more
Walking away with new experiences
        Wanted or not
        Welcomed

We Learn
    Grow
        Grieve
            Laugh
                Lose
                    Love
                        Reflect

Reflection

Unaware then what 52 weeks could bring.

Sitting in silence with pen to paper.

Recording a year as it unfolds.

Through the seasons of life, love,
death, emotions we write.

The pages staring back
at us now, a yearbook of life.

Wishes, what-ifs, victories, losses
documented now.

We find our voices, one week at a time.

We are here, we always were.

But now, we believe. What is
capable within us

I turn the page
                Blank
                              Again.

Reminded of the gift
   That is
            Time.
The privilege to Write,
Improve, Reflect, Rejoice.

We come together
yet again.
The community created on Words,
Vulnerability, and Love.

We will cherish
What we created
The gift to ourselves

The authors were always in us.
But now the mirror we were
looking in
finally
lifting its fog –

Enough for us to see ourselves
For what we are
what we always were.
Humans trying to process life
as it unfolds in front of us.

We will continue to turn to the blank pages.

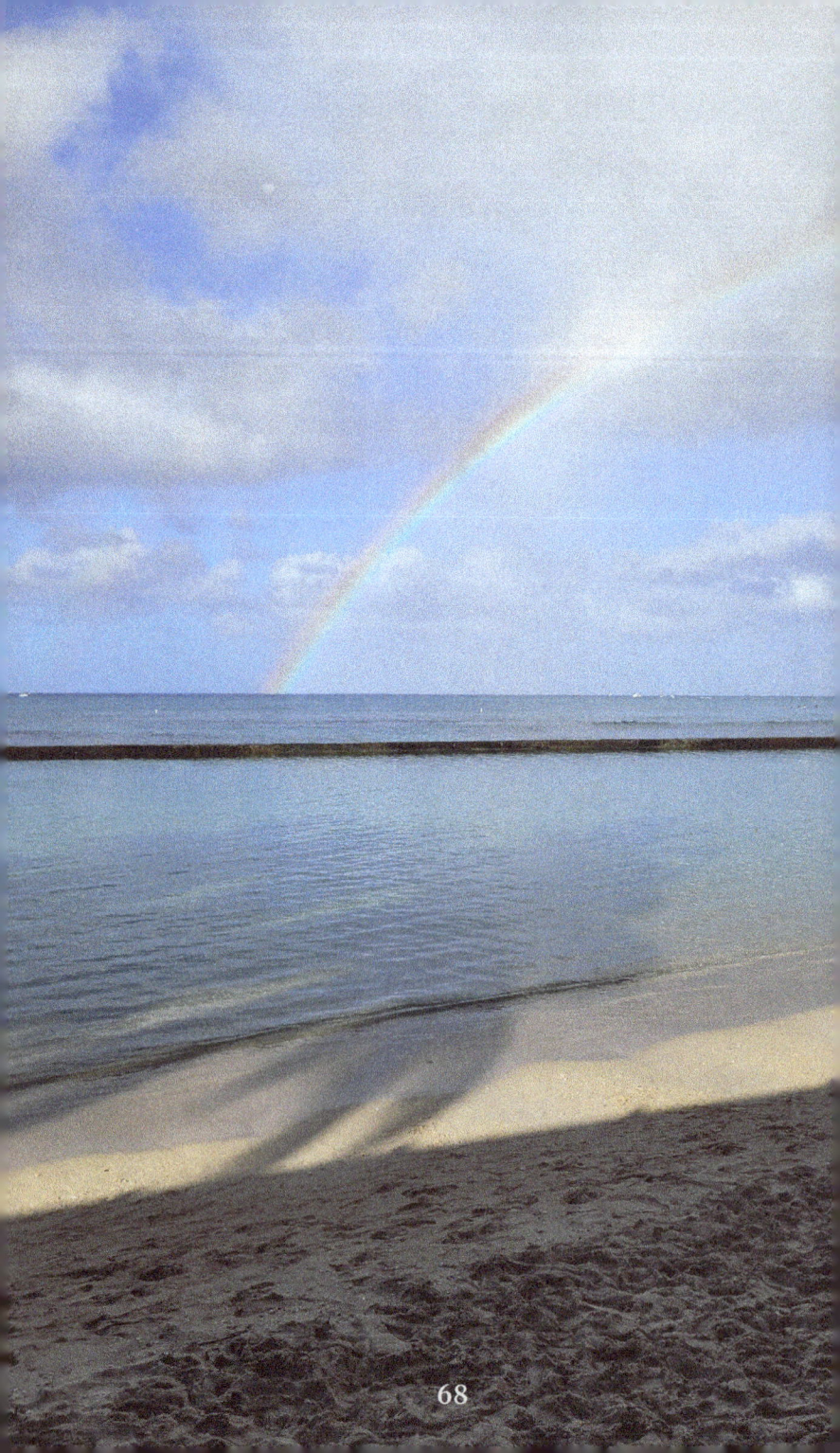

Life is Hard and Beautiful

May you find peace in knowing they can coexist

Dear Younger Self

Dear Younger Self,

I wish I could have told you:
hold on for the wild ride,
focus on the joy.

Remember, you are not a statistic.

Rather than focusing on the sand
draining from the hourglass

look up and enjoy the sunset in front of you.

Time Stamped Moments

Lean in
Look back
at the
Time Stamped Moments
of your life

Those seconds
that felt like
an eternity

You were a speck as
you felt the universe swirling

Imprinting a new chapter
on your life's book

What did those
Time Stamped Moments
teach you then?

What could you learn
from them now?

Time Stamped Moments
Here to show us the way
A knowing deep inside
If we take the time
To hear
A Calling

Story

I hope someday she recognizes
The magic of our story

She can't see now
What these appointments mean
It's her day off from school
But my day at the clinic
She tags along as she has so many times before

As she grows older
She cringes more
When she sees the needles

I cringe
As I think of all my story
Has exposed her to

We make the best of our time there
Just like we try to do with each day we're given
We take on the villains together
And embrace the happily ever after
We have right now

I hope someday
She too
Recognizes
The magic of our story.

Story: Part 2

Some day you'll recognize
    The magic of our story

Remember Disney World?
    We have magic like that too.
We are princesses living
    With our Prince – Daddy.
We are powerful brave and strong
    Like Lady Bug!
Sometimes we might feel like
    Mirabel — searching for
    Our power.

But some day you'll recognize
    The magic of our story.

You join me today
    You lead the way
You bring joy
    To the nurses
You bring joy to me every day.

Living Room

The house that was built
    For dreams to fill
Quickly changed to lost hope

After twelve-hour work days
I'd sit with the thoughts about
All I was robbed of
No answers
Just the darkness
Of what was not

Then, we let others in
Dreamed again of what could be
In no time at all
    Our perfect surrogate
    Surely sent from above
Appointments, drives, procedures, scares

The same living room, once dark
Now filled with newborn cries

It was also this room
Where I took the call
That changed it all

Now, added to the newborn cries
Were Mommy tears of what might never be

Next toddler tantrums
With a woman too overwhelmed
By all that life is
And is not
Emotions uncontrolled
Pent up until there's nowhere to go

In this room
Dance parties express what words cannot

School age now
Cuddling on the couch and dissecting the day

Barbie dolls strewn about
Big Dreams inside the little pink house

Suddenly the room is filled
With play dates and fun

Another blink of the eyes
Silence again

Like the days when dreams were lost

But this time
Silence only during school hours
The Barbie Dreamhouse staring back at me

While I await the one who made it all
A Reality

Touch

I hold her hands
We know she's slowly slipping away

The independent, strong one
The one that hates hugs

—

She now reaches for my hands
For my vulnerability tied to her own
For the sisterly love
That we always knew was between us

I want to hold on forever
I want my love to strengthen her
If even just for a few more hours
For one more conversation with her daughters

I arrive home

She runs towards me
Expressing her pure joy

"Mommy! You're Home. I missed you!"

My arms are open
It's as if I'm witnessing her smile
For the very first time
As I cling tight
Her words immediately bring tears of peace

"You smell like Auntie."

I hold her
While silently thanking my best friend
– my soul sister –
For all that she's been

And still is

Overwhelmed

Overwhelmed. I'm not sure how I will do this.
What do I focus on next?
I know I should take action, but
it feels too big. So I sit. I flounder.
I let it build inside me until
I feel it in my tight muscles.

I know I must create. Do. Move.
Brain-dump, create lists, start tiny, chisel away
until the stone is a carving, is art.

It was art all along.

All
    steps
        were
            necessary.

Overwhelmed Reframed

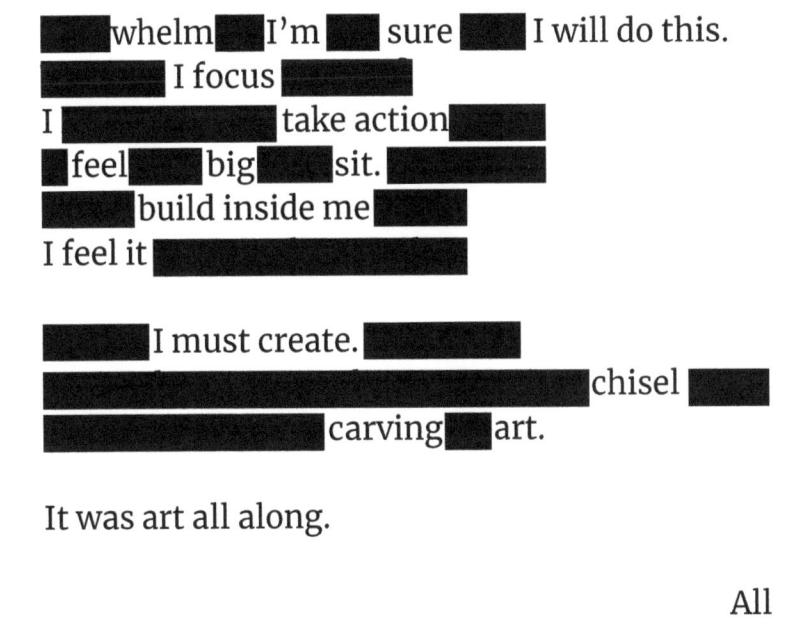

▇ whelm ▇ I'm ▇ sure ▇ I will do this.
▇ I focus ▇
I ▇ take action ▇
▇ feel ▇ big ▇ sit. ▇
▇ build inside me ▇
I feel it ▇

▇ I must create. ▇
▇ chisel ▇
▇ carving ▇ art.

It was art all along.

                                          All
                               steps
                        were
            necessary.

Belong

I once belonged to my corporate career.
At one time to my cancer diagnosis.
For far too long I let fear hold me hostage.
That was then.
So, what *do* I belong to now?

I belong amongst the stars.
Amongst the trees and forest.
Amongst the vast plains
and the open, rough seas.

I belong to the wind,
to which I feel, these days,
is leading me more
than the ground under my feet.

I belong to my family,
to the ones that hold me,
to the ones I hold tight.

I belong to my heart. To my joy.

To what do I belong?
It's not a Who, Where, Why.
To what do I belong?

I belong to the beauty I put into the world.
I belong to my art, to these words.

Even In

Even in times of darkness
may you still notice the beauty

Even in times of question
may you still hold on to hope

Even in times of weary
may you turn to faith for
strength you don't think you have

Even in times of deep sorrow
may you remember a story
to give you a reason to smile

Even after your loved ones leave this earth
may you find comfort knowing
they're still with you

Even when you are hurting
may you find your people
your community
those who will hold you up

Authentic

A word chosen for the year
    to be real, raw, honest.

To let go of what's no longer serving me,
to trust,
    on all levels
that the answer is authenticity.

To trust
that authenticity
    is the universe
    inspiring me
    to show up,
    to give and receive energy, light, love.

Unaware then
    just what authenticity
    would entail.

Serving, mentoring, saying goodbye
    to a career,
so I could say my last goodbyes
    to my soul sister.

Being stripped of so much. Yet,
    what was left was
    what I was meant to find –
my authentic self.

Expectation

It lets us down
It keeps us anxious and scared

We worry
   about what's to come
We disappoint ourselves
   when something doesn't go as planned

Instead of living in the moment,
we forecast what will happen;

Often left upset when reality
doesn't match our illusion.

What if...
   What if we were to let go of expectations?

What if we were to let go of the extra weight
   we put on ourselves
   and instead
   just
      enjoyed
           what is?

What if...
   life was better than our expectations,

   because we decided it could be?

Writing

I set out to write
so that my daughter would remember
who I was,
as I lived in fear of not being here
to watch her grow up.

Over time,
the intention of my writing morphed.

I was no longer writing
so my daughter would know me
I was writing
so I could know myself.

As the years carried on
writing carried me.

I healed from the trauma my body endured
from cancer;
my fear of dying changed to joyfully living.

I broke down the bricks, one by one.
I dismantled the wall I had built around myself.

My heart softened.
And I finally let go of who I thought I had to be.
And started living for who I wanted to be.

The Timeless Moment

I want to protect the fragility that it is.
But can I, really? I want to warn others.
But their experiences are different
than my own. There's a freedom in
letting go. Once I give up control,
only then can I enjoy the moment
that is this minute
this hour.
I needed to
destroy the gripping
I was holding so tightly to. The sand
will flow whether contained or not.
To sparkle on I must accept what is.
With those I love the most, the sun
shines on us. We sparkle together.
I know I'll hold this moment in time.

What Matters

When the sand runs out

It's not the car I drove
Or the stuff I collected

It's not the money left in my bank account
Or the jobs I clocked into
Or the titles I was given

It's not the fear I had about
    how I was perceived
    how I looked
    flying
    failing
    loving
    death

      No, in the end, my fear
          will not have mattered.

What matters in the end
Is that I found meaning
    in a day,
    in an image,
    in even a tiny part of my story

What matters in the end
Is if I was able to
    forgive
    apologize
    let go
    accept

What matters in the end

Is how I showed up
For myself
For others
How I lived with
love, grace, and inner strength

Dear Cancer,

You tried to ruin me. My body.
My trust in the future.
You tried to tear apart our marriage
strip our opportunity of becoming parents.

But you did not — you will not — win.

You tried so hard to take so much.
But I gained more from you,
than you took from me.

I won't say I'm grateful we met.
But knowing you since age 27
you helped me grow, learn, and
live life differently.

Because of you
I lost my hair, my breasts, my fertility,
my open communication with loved ones.

Because of you
I went through menopause before celebrating
my 30th birthday.
15 years later, I still have the scars from
radiation and surgery.

But
also because of you
I met some of my best friends.
I experienced unconditional love.

Because of you
I chased my dreams and became a mommy,
I learned to trust my body again,
I learned to trust God through all things,
I found my authentic self.

Because of you, I learned
what really matters in the end.

Best Regards,

    Jonell
    Metastatic Breast Cancer Thriver

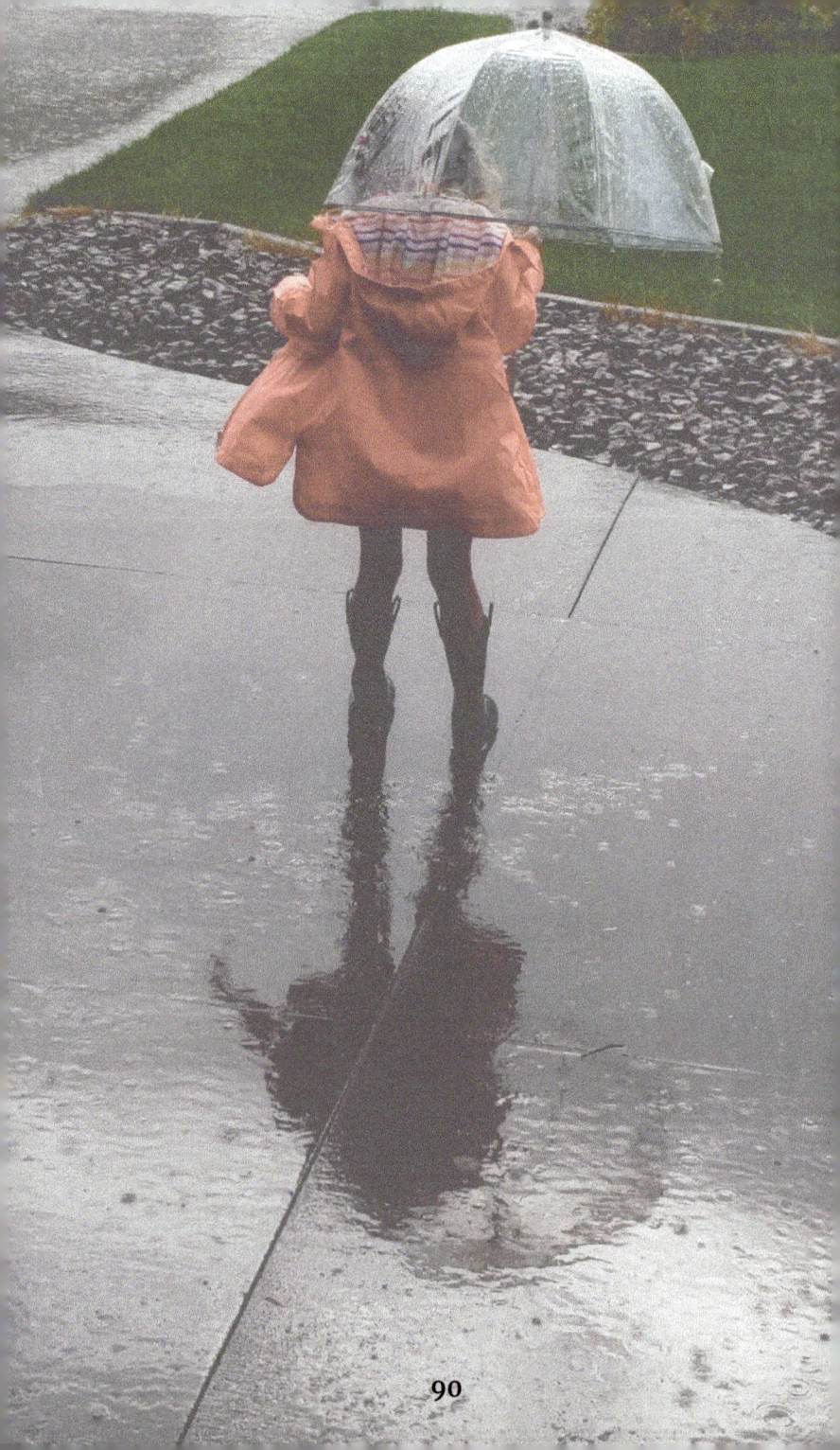

Reflect and Write

*Prompts and space for you,
should you feel inspired
to put pen to paper*

Let yourself be. Write whatever is on your mind: your grocery list, your fears, your excitement, anything.

Think of a place you love to hang out. Write about the sights, sounds, smells, and feelings you have while there.

Did you learn anything about yourself from these poems or any other writing that has significance to you?

Set a timer for 7 minutes and write anything that comes to mind about the word 'grief'.

Set a timer for 7 minutes and write anything that comes to mind about the word 'joy'.

Think of a hard time in your life. Try to find a dash of beauty within the experience. Write about both.

Spend 5 minutes writing about a hard time. Next, use the "Overwhelmed Reframed" poem on page 79 as inspiration, and black out the negative words in your own work. Finally, reflect on how that made you feel.

Acknowledgments

Seeing my first published book enter the world was hard and beautiful. It's a dream and calling that has been on my heart for years. This process took many people believing in me, before I believed in myself. Saying thank you will never be enough.

To my rock, my groom: having you by my side through life is the best gift I have been given. Thank you for holding me through the fear, anxiety, and overwhelm of life. I can't wait to continue to build our lives together.

To my miracle baby: it's because of you that my faith was restored. You taught me that big dreams can come true. I thank God daily that I get to continue to watch you grow. My hope for you is that you always live life as joyfully as you do now.

To my parents: the ones who have cheered me on, even before 2nd grade when I was too scared to swing the softball bat. Thank you for your unending support, through the hard times and the beautiful times. Thank you for showing me what love and faith look like.

To my extended family and friends: thank you for reading and commenting on my updates as I took on all my cancer treatments. Your comments kept me going and calmed me when fear crept in.

To my Survivor Sisters, the ones we had to say goodbye to all too soon, and the ones who continue to walk beside me on Earth: because of the space you provided, I was able to be honest about the hard moments in life.

To Joanne: thank you for showing me the power of words and how to process my trauma through writing. Thank you for creating a community of writers within which I felt seen, heard, and loved.

To 49th Parallel: I love that we have each other for inspiration and accountability. Having you to process the hard times has helped me see the beauty sprinkled within.

To Jennifer: your feedback, suggestions, creative ideas, and editing of this book was invaluable. I know this book is stronger because of your time and passionate professionalism.

To my author friends: every book you published showed me what was possible and what dream I held close to my heart.

To my God, my Creator, my Protector: thank you for your patience as I built true faith in you, one area of life at a time. Thank you for using the hard times I endured to show me the beautiful gifts I hold. I know you are walking with me and my family, no matter what.

Thank You

My hope is that putting this book into the world might help you to to heal, grow, or see life from a new perspective.

I would love to hear what resonated with you. Please reach out to me at:

      janellmeier@gmail.com

If you'd like to see what else I'm up to you can connect with me at my website:

      janellmeier.com

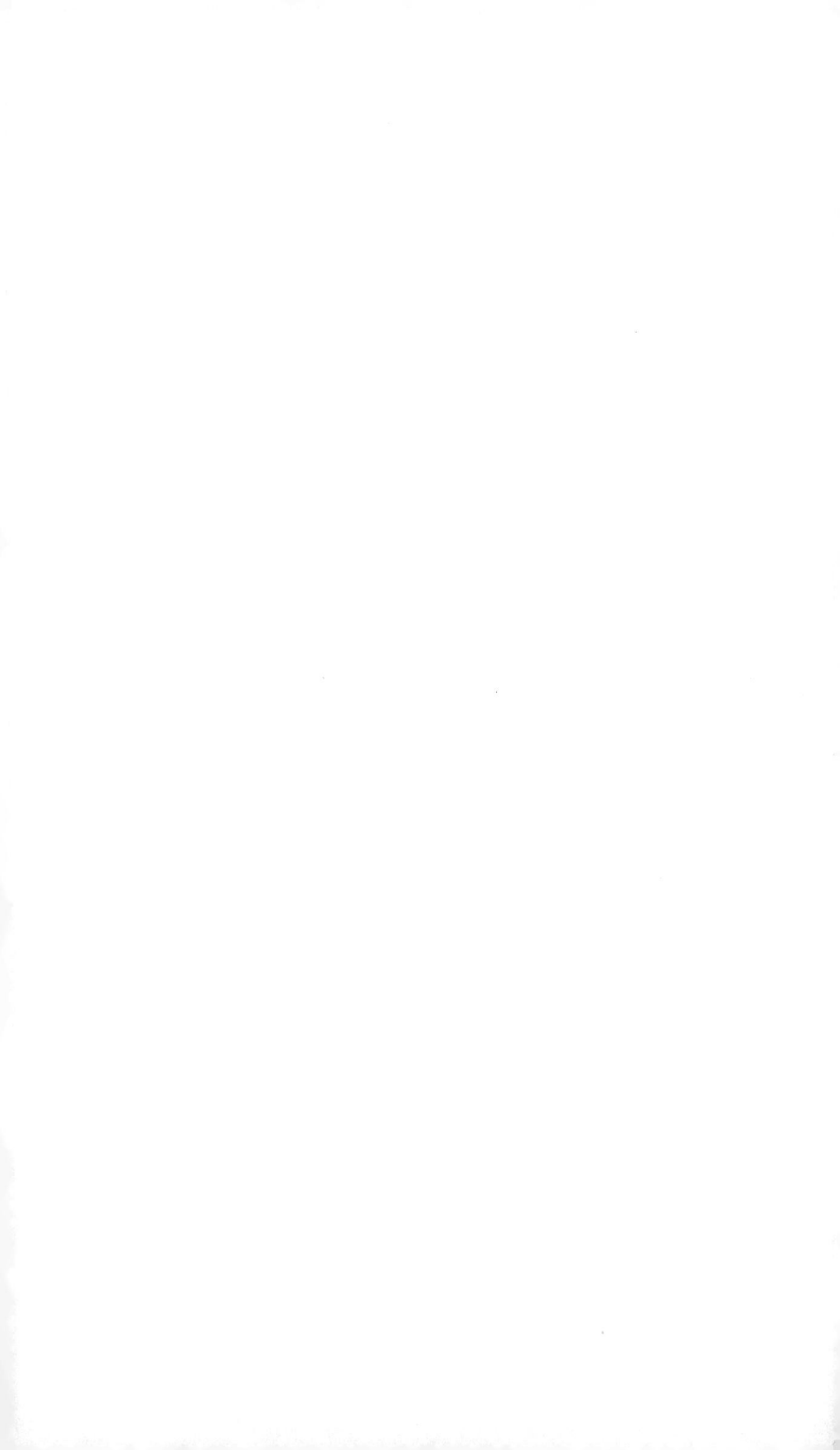